# Lectin-Free Acid Reflux Diet

The Proven Diet For Heartburn, Indigestion and Bariatric Patients Following Weight Loss Surgery - With Kent McCabe Emma Aqiyl Susan Frazier

Tim Shepherd

Lactin S. Campbell

Kent McCabe

# Table of Contents

# Introduction

Imagine how it would feel finally being free of pain, being free of inflammation, and being free of many of the ailments and diseases that you suffer from each day. Maybe you have tried a wide variety of medications to help. Maybe you have tried every holistic approach, but nothing seems to work.

The solution that you need may be as simple as changing up the diet that you follow. By changing up the diet so it doesn't include foods that are high in lectin, you can reduce inflammation and other issues in your body. This guidebook will help you get started by looking at what lectin is, why it is such a bad thing, and some of the foods that you can avoid to ensure lectin doesn't cause any more problems for you.

In addition to learning a bit about lectin and some of the benefits of following this kind of diet plan, we will also look at some of the recipes you can add to your life to keep you happy and healthy. Reducing lectin doesn't have to be a chore, but you will be amazed by the difference you see once you start, and this guidebook is the tool you need to get that done.

When you are ready to finally get rid of some of the pain and intestinal problems you are dealing with and you want a safe and effective solution, then make sure to read through this guidebook to help you get started

# PART 1

# Chapter 1: What is the Lectin-free Diet?

The lectin-free diet is one that asks the follower to try and eliminate all, or the majority, of the lectins that they consume in their meals. Basically, the lectins are a type of protein that will bind carbs together in the body. They will then stick to the membranes of your cells inside your stomach, causing issues with your digestion and how well it can work. It can even affect how well you feel each day.

These lectins are going to be found in many foods you eat, including plant and animal products. However, they are found in the highest amounts in legumes, nightshade vegetables, dairy products, and even grains. Some are toxic, such as ricin, and others are not considered as bad for your health. Even the non-toxic ones are able to cause some issues to your health and well-being though.

The point of the lectin-free diet is to help you learn more about lectins so you can understand why they are so bad and you can choose to limit them in your diet. The lectin-free diet helps you to reduce foods that are high in lectins from your diet, including some of your favorites, in order to help you feel healthier overall. It isn't as restrictive as some diet plans and you will still have many options to choose from with this eating plan, but you will need to cut out a few things.

You will find that there is a good deal of benefits that come from this diet plan. It is known to help your digestion, it can clear up health issues like irritable bowel syndrome, and it can even help you lose weight if you combine it with a low-calorie diet as well. Lack of energy, brain fog, extra inflammation throughout the body, and more can also be helped when you go on a lectin-free diet plan.

## Where are lectins found?

Lectins can be found in many of the foods that you enjoy today. They are found in higher amounts in foods like grains and raw legumes. Many people who deal with issues from inflammation will choose to cut out lectins, which means they are going to need to avoid foods like grains, anything that has gluten in it, legumes, peanuts, and even some vegetables to get relief.

## Why are lectins bad for me?

Humans can run into trouble digesting most lectins. In fact, these can be resistant to the enzymes in the stomach, and the lectins can make it all the way through the stomach without any changes. In addition, lectins can be very sticky and this makes them more prone to attaching to the walls of your intestines. Once the lectins reach the intestines, they are able to disrupt the routine maintenance of the cells, so the wear and tear that naturally occurs there is just going to get worse.

This is the main reason why consuming a large number of lectins in your diet can end up causing issues like digestive distress. Repeated exposure to lectins can end up causing damage to the wall of your stomach. Substances that are unwanted can find their way through the wall and then enter into the bloodstream in a process that is known as leaky gut.

When the lectins begin to leak into the bloodstream, they can interact with various things, including the antibodies. These antibodies are the core component of your immune system, and it won't take long until you have an immune reaction against the lectins, as well as against any tissues in the body that the lectins may have bound themselves too.

There are a lot of negatives that come with eating too many lectins in your diet. While having a few on occasion isn't that big of a deal, some of the negatives that you should watch out for will include:

- Lectins are hard for the stomach to digest.
- These lectins have the ability to cause some damage to the wall of your stomach and intestines, which can lead to leaky gut syndrome.
- These lectins are known to act like an anti-nutrient.
- These lectins are going to interfere with your digestion and how well you are able to absorb foods.
- If these lectin levels get too high, you could run into issues with nutritional deficiencies.
- While more information is needed, it is believed that these lectins could be responsible for several different autoimmune conditions including rheumatoid arthritis.
- These lectins have the ability to upset your digestion, which could lead to lectin poisoning as well as gastroenteritis.

Because of these reasons and more, it is often recommended that people stay away from foods that have a high amount of lectin. And if you suffer from some autoimmune diseases, irritable bowel syndrome, and other issues with your stomach or intestines, it may be worth your time to look at a lectin-free diet and see if it can provide you some relief.

There are some benefits that come with consuming lectins, such as helping with the immune and helping regulate cell adhesion, but this is only when you eat them in smaller amounts. Considering many of the foods that are high in lectin are common in the American diet and are eaten in high amounts, many of these benefits are counteracted and reduced. It is often better to reduce the number of lectins that are consumed to help get the intestines and the stomach happy.

## Top Foods that have Lectin in Them

There are a lot of foods that contain lectin in them. Many of these foods are considered nutritious so you may already be consuming them without realizing that you are causing harm to the gut. Although you are able to find some lectins in many of the foods that you eat, some of the places where lectin content seems to be really high include:

- Peanuts
- Tomatoes
- Peas
- Red kidney beans
- Wheat germ
- Peppers
- Lentils
- Soybeans
- Eggplant
- Potatoes

It is important that when you go on the lectin-free diet, you learn how to avoid these types of foods as much as possible. They are going to increase the amount of lectin that is found in your body and can make the health conditions worse than before.

## Can I reduce the number of lectins in my diet?

It is pretty easy to reduce the number of lectins in your diet if you know the basics and you take the right precautions. Eliminating foods that have high levels of lectin in them can be the first step. Cooking your food can help to get rid of a lot of lectins, such as in the case of soybeans and other legumes. Soaking and fermenting can help aid this as well.

Reducing the number of lectins in your diet can make a big difference in how healthy you feel and it can be as easy as cutting out a few types of foods and cooking any that you do decide to add into your diet. Fermenting some of your foods can be a unique way to change up some of the meals that you enjoy while still getting rid of those harmful lectins before they can cause more damage to your intestines and cause an autoimmune response in your body.

## What are the benefits of a lectin-free diet?

Lectins are in many of the foods that we eat, but many times, we don't even realize we are sick. We have gotten so used to the way that we feel that it seems normal. When you go on the lectin-free diet, it won't take long until you start to notice a big difference. Some of the health benefits that you will notice with this kind of diet plan include:

- Helps fight off sensitivities to some foods

- Helps you to avoid toxic foods
- Can protect the digestive tract
- In some people, it will reduce the number and the risk for ulcers.
- Can assist in losing weight
- Reduces brain fog

## Is cooking important on this diet?

Yes, cooking your food is very important when it comes to the lectin-free diet. You should not eat many foods raw, except maybe a few fresh fruits and vegetables. Many of the food products that you consume on a regular basis will contain at least a small amount of lectin. But when you choose to cook up these foods, you are able to eliminate most, if not all, of the lectin that is found inside of those foods.

This is great news for those who are taking a look at the food list for the lectin diet and feel worried about what they will to eat. You will be able to add a lot of these foods back onto your diet, at least in small amounts, when you make sure to cook them properly. And if you are just looking to reduce the lectins you consume, then cooking is going to be your best friend to get that number as low as possible.

There are a lot of different cooking methods that work in order to help you stick with the lectin-free diet. Many people like to work with the pressure cooker because it uses really high temperatures and pressure to cook the food you want to eat. And with those high temperatures, it is easier to reduce the amount of lectin that is found in your food.

# Chapter 2: What Should I Eat on a Lectin-Free Diet?

When you are on a lectin-free diet, you need to make sure that you are careful with the foods you eat. You will need to eliminate some of the foods that you enjoyed before to make sure that you limit your lectin intake as much as possible. This chapter will explore some of the foods that you can eat, and some of the ones you should avoid when you are ready to start out on the lectin-free diet plan.

## Foods That You Should Avoid

To keep things simple, you want to avoid any foods that contain high amounts of lectin in them. This helps you to avoid inflammation, autoimmune responses, and issues with leaky gut. We will split up our foods into two groups. The first one is going to be foods that you can have, but it is best to limit them as much as you can. They aren't the worst, but eating them in really high amounts, or if you are really sensitive to lectins, can make the matter worse.

The second list includes foods that you should avoid at all costs. It is best to never eat these when you are on a lectin-free diet or limit them to once or twice a year at most. These have really high levels of lectin in them that can make you sick.

The first group of foods, the ones that you should try to limit in your diet, includes:

- Grains. If you do decide to go with grains or products that are made out of grains, go with white flour rather than with wheat.

- Fruit. You can have some in-season fruit as long as you keep the consumption down to a minimum.

- Be careful with the nightshade vegetables. This includes options like tomatoes, potatoes, peppers, and eggplants. You can enjoy tomatoes on occasion as long as they are cooked properly.

- Squash

- Be careful of the legumes. This includes the peanuts, lentils, peas, and beans. You can add these a bit to the diet, but do not rely on soaking them before eating. Make sure they are all cooked properly to avoid as many lectins as possible.

Then, you will also need to watch for the second group of foods. These are foods that you must avoid completely on this kind of diet because they have a ton of lectin and can pretty much ruin all the progress you are trying to make. Some of the foods that you must avoid on a lectin-free diet include:

- A1 Milk

- Any meat that comes from an animal that was corn-fed. You can still eat meat, but make sure that they are pasture-raised rather than ones that are corn-fed.

- Corn

These foods can be really bad for your health and will often cause complications like what we have talked about before. Eating them can cause lectins to build up in your system. While some of them are a bit lower in lectins than other foods, it is still important that you avoid them as much as possible for the health of your stomach.

## Foods That You Can Enjoy On A Lectin-Free Diet

Now that we have taken a look at some of the foods that you need to avoid because they are high in lectin content, it is time to look at some of the foods that you don't need to avoid on this diet plan. There are lots of health and delicious foods that you can enjoy because they don't contain a lot of lectin in them. Eating a diet that is full of variety and lots of healthy and wholesome foods can be your best bet on this eating plan. Some of the foods that you can enjoy will include the following:

- Fruits in small amounts: Pick out options that are in season to avoid lectins as much as possible. These do contain some lectins so you may need to limit them a bit.
- Meats: As long as the meat is pasture-raised, it is fine to enjoy it. Go for some healthy options like beef, turkey, and chicken.
- A2 milk
- Sweet potatoes can be consumed, but take the time to cook them first.
- Leafy and green vegetables
- All cruciferous vegetables. These are broccoli, sprouts, and more.
- Asparagus
- Garlic
- Onion
- Celery
- Mushrooms
- Avocado

- Olive oil

- Olives

The foods on this list can be enjoyed as much as you want with your meals. They will provide you with lots of energy and even the nutrients your body needs to heal after too many lectins. Try to fill your plate with as much variety as you can to ensure you get the most nutrition possible. You can also occasionally pair them up with some of the not allowed foods to add in a bit more variety when needed.

When you first get started on this diet plan, take the time to write down this list and take it to the grocery store with you. Then, when you are uncertain about whether a food fits in with this new diet plan or not, you can pull out this list and double check. You can also do the same thing when you are looking for new recipes to try. Even if the recipe is not in a lectin-free cookbook, you can look over the list and see if one of your old favorites will fit in.

Luckily, this guidebook will contain a ton of great recipes that will work on the lectin-free diet, so you are able to get healthy, without having to do all the work.

# Chapter 3: Exercising and the Lectin-free diet

While you are on the lectin-free diet, it is a good idea to include some exercise. This can help you to burn more calories to lose weight, can make you feel good, and can speed up the recovery process. If you have never done much exercise, it is important to start out slowly. But over time, you can increase the exercise and see even better results.

There are many different types of workouts that you can choose to do when you go on a lectin-free diet. Mixing the different workouts together can ensure that you get the most health benefits, but remember that a workout you will stick with for the long term is always the best option. Some of the choices that you can make when it comes to the type of exercise you want to do include the following:

## Cardio

Cardio is a great option to go with when you want to burn calories quickly and get that heart working a bit better. It is a very effective way to lean up and lose weight and there are a lot of options with this. You can choose to do walking or running, swimming, dancing, biking, and more to help you get the benefits from cardio exercise.

It is a good idea to spend at least a few days a week getting some form of cardio exercise and you can mix up the workouts to ensure that you get something new each day and you don't start to feel bored.

Another option to try out is HIIT. This is high-intensity interval training. You will do your workout at a regular intensity that you are used to. Then throughout the workout, you will add in short bursts, usually between twenty to thirty seconds, of higher intensity. So, if you are walking, you would do a fast pace and then do a full out sprint for twenty to thirty seconds a few times through the workout. This can make the workout more efficient and can help you to gain more endurance while getting your workout done in less time than before.

## Weightlifting

If you go on the lectin-free diet in the hopes of losing weight, then you may want to include a few days of weight lifting into your schedule. Many people are scared of starting a strength training program because they don't want to gain bulky muscles or they think it is too hard. But just adding a few weights to your week, you can get lean muscles without to much work.

Start out slowly when you do a weight training program. Just do what you are comfortable with and slowly build up to more. Some workout programs will allow you to combine together your weight training with some cardio and those can be great options as well.

## Stretching and Flexibility

It is a good idea to spend a little bit of time doing some stretching and flexibility during the week. You can consider doing a few minutes each day if you would like or do some longer sessions once or twice a week. This could include just some basic stretching or some yoga to help reduce stress and relax the whole body.

These stretching exercises can be nice because they give you a break from some of the other workouts that you do. They are also good for reducing the amount of stress your muscles and joints feel and can prevent injuries when you do the other exercises so you can stay safe and feel great.

Mixing up these workouts can be a great option to help you get all the benefits possible. But if you prefer one type of workout over another, it is fine to spend some time working on that one. It is always better to do that workout if you stick with it than to not do any workout at all.

# Chapter 4: Tips to Make the Lectin-Free Diet Easier

A lectin-free diet is not one that is supposed to be really difficult for you to follow. Yes, you will need to make some changes in what you eat on a daily basis, but it can be really effective at helping you with a bunch of health conditions and helping you to feel better. But there may be times when you want to indulge or you feel it is too hard to stick on this diet plan. Some of the tips that you can follow to make the lectin-free diet easier include:

- Use a pressure cooker: The high temperatures that are in a pressure cooker can be great for reducing lectin levels in food, plus it helps you to get meals done quickly.

- Eat some extra fiber: Since you are cutting out some vegetables and legumes, it can be a bit more difficult to get enough fiber into your diet. Consider adding in a dietary supplement to help you get enough fiber. Or eat enough vegetables and fruits to help you get the fiber that you need.

- Find someone to do the diet with you: Going on a diet plan alone can be hard. If you can find someone else to do it with you, you will have someone to support you, someone to be on your side, and someone there to encourage you along the way.

- Take out one food at a time: If you are worried about getting started on the lectin-free diet, you may want to consider taking one food from the list out of your diet at a time. This can still get you to the same end result, even if it takes longer, and can make it a bit easier for you to accomplish.

- See what works the best for you. Some people find that they are really sensitive to foods that have lectin in them. If this is true to you, then it is best to just reduce all the lectin-containing products that you have. But for others, you may want to experiment with just taking out one food at a time and see what works the best with you.

The lectin diet can be a great option to help you to get rid of some common health concerns simply by taking a few types of foods out of your diet. By following some of the tips above, you will be able to get the most benefits out of this diet plan without any trouble at all!

# Chapter 5: Lectin-Free Diet Breakfast Delights

## Nutty Oatmeal

**What's inside:**

- Blueberries (.5 c.)
- Ground nutmeg (.25 tsp.)
- Cinnamon (1 tsp.)
- Diced avocado (1)
- Stevia (2 Tbsp.)
- Sliced almonds (.5 c.)
- Chopped pecans (.5 c.)
- Shredded coconut (1 c.)
- Coconut milk (1 c.)
- Coconut oil (1 Tbsp.)

**How to make:**

1. Take out the inner pot of the slow cooker and grease it with some coconut oil. Place it back inside.
2. Add in the nutmeg, cinnamon, stevia, avocado, almonds, pecans, coconut, and coconut milk to the slow cooker.
3. Add the lid to the top and cook on a low setting for eight hours.
4. Top the oatmeal with some blueberries and then enjoy.

# Sausage Meatloaf

## What's inside:

- Mashed banana (1 c.)
- Salt (.5 tsp.)
- Pepper
- Fennel seeds (1 tsp.)
- Dried thyme (1 tsp.)
- Dried oregano (2 tsp.)
- Garlic, minced (2 tsp.)
- Almond flour (.5 c.)
- Chopped sweet onion (1)
- Ground pork (2 lbs.)
- Olive oil (1 Tbsp.)

## How to make:

1. Use some olive oil to grease the inside of the slow cooker.
2. Bring out a bowl and mix together the salt, pepper, fennel seeds, thyme, garlic, oregano, almond flour, banana, onion, and pork.
3. Pour this mixture into the slow cooker and form it into a loaf. Make sure there is about half an inch on all sides of the meat.
4. Place the lid on top of this mixture and cover it up. Cook on a low setting until the meat is cooked through.
5. After this time, slice up the meatloaf before serving.

# Creamy Broccoli Casserole

## What's inside:

- Cashew cream (1.5 c.)
- Pepper
- Ground nutmeg (.5 tsp.)
- Coconut milk (2 c.)
- Almond flour (.25 c.)
- Cauliflower (1 lb.)
- Broccoli (1 lb.)
- Olive oil (1 Tbsp.)

## How to make:

1. Grease the slow cooker with some olive oil. Then add the prepared cauliflower and broccoli inside.
2. Take out a bowl so that you can stir together a cup of the cashew cream with the pepper, coconut milk, and almond flour.
3. Pour this mixture over the vegetables and then add the rest of the cashew cream on top.
4. Cover up the slow cooker and cook on a low setting for six hours before serving.

# Healthy Granola

**What's inside:**

- Salt (.25 tsp.)
- Nutmeg, ground (.25 tsp.)
- Cinnamon (.5 tsp.)
- Stevia (2 Tbsp.)
- Slivered almonds (.5 c.)
- Hazelnuts (.5 c.)
- Shredded coconut (1 c.)
- Sunflower seeds (1 c.)
- Chopped pecans (1 c.)
- Maple extract (1 tsp.)
- Vanilla (2 tsp.)
- Coconut oil (.5 c.)

**How to make:**

1. Take out a bowl and combine together the vanilla, maple, and oil. Stir it well before adding in the salt, cinnamon, nutmeg, stevia, almonds, hazelnuts, sunflower seeds, coconut, and pecans.
2. Toss these ingredients together well before moving over to the slow cooker.
3. Add the lid on top and cook these ingredients on a low setting for three hours.
4. Move the granola over to a baking sheet and then cover up with foil. Allow the granola a time to cool down before serving for supper.

# Chapter 6: Chicken and Poultry Dishes

## Chicken Taco Dish

### What's inside:

- Taco seasoning (3 Tbsp.)
- Chicken broth (1 c.)
- Chicken breast (1 lb.)

### How to make:

1. Take out a bowl and mix together the broth and the taco seasoning.

2. Prepare the slow cooker and then add the chicken breasts inside. Pour the broth mixture on top of the chicken.

3. Place the lid on top of the chicken and then let it cook on a medium setting for six hours.

4. After this time is up, turn the heat off and let the chicken set for a few minutes. Take the lid off and use a fork to shred the chicken.

5. Serve the chicken with some sweet potatoes and your chosen sauce.

# Mushroom and Bacon Chicken

## What's inside:

- Coconut cream (1 c.)
- Chopped thyme (2 tsp.)
- Chicken broth (.5 c.)
- Garlic, minced (1 Tbsp.)
- Diced onion (1 sweet)
- Quartered button mushrooms (2 c.)
- Chicken (2 lbs.)
- Diced bacon (.25 lb.)
- Coconut oil (3 Tbsp.)

## How to make:

1. Take out a skillet and warm it up on the stove. Add in a few tablespoons of oil and give the oil time to warm up in the skillet.
2. When the oil is warm, add in the bacon and let it cook until it reaches the doneness level that you like. Move the bacon over to a plate and set to the side.
3. Add your chicken to this skillet and let it brown for five minutes. Then move the chicken over to the slow cooker before topping with the thyme, broth, onion, garlic, and mushrooms.
4. Cover up the slow cooker and cook this mixture on a low setting for seven to eight hours.
5. After this time, stir in your coconut cream before serving.

# Duck Roast

## What's inside:

- Cubed sweet potatoes (1.5 c)
- Chicken broth (1.5 c.)
- Onion (1)
- Duck roast (2 lbs.)
- Dry vegetable soup mix (1 pack)

## How to make:

1. Add the duck roast to the inside of the slow cooker.
2. Take out a bowl and blend together the chicken broth and the soup mix.
3. Slice up the onion into quarters and then move those along with the sweet potatoes into the slow cooker, arranging them around the chicken.
4. Pour the soup mix over everything and then place the lid on top of the slow cooker.
5. Cook this mixture on a high setting for two hours. After the time is up, let the meat sit for a bit and then serve warm.

# Lettuce Chicken Wraps

## What's inside:

- Swiss chard leaves for wraps
- Pepper
- Salt
- Red pepper flakes (.25 tsp.)
- Ground ginger
- Coconut aminos (.33 c)
- Crushed pineapple (8 oz.)
- Minced garlic cloves (3)
- Diced onion (.5)
- Chicken thighs (.5 lbs.)
- Chicken breast (1 lb.)

## How to make:

1. Add the garlic, chicken, and onion to the slow cooker.
2. Take out a bowl and combine together the pepper, salt, red pepper flakes, coconut aminos, lime juice, and pineapple.
3. Stir this well and combine to the slow cooker. Stir well and cook on a low setting for about four hours.
4. After this time, take the chicken out and shred it up with a fork. Return the chicken to the slow cooker.
5. Assemble the wraps by laying out the lettuce leaves and adding some of the chicken mixture on top before serving.

# Turkey Legs

## What's inside:

- Chopped parsley (2 Tbsp.)
- Chicken broth (.5 c.)
- Poultry seasoning (2 tsp.)
- Dried thyme (1 Tbsp.)
- pepper
- salt
- turkey legs (2 lbs.)
- olive oil (3 Tbsp.)

## How to make:

1. Take out a skillet and let it warm up with a few tablespoons of olive oil on the stove.
2. Season your turkey with some pepper and salt along with the poultry seasoning and the thyme.
3. Add the turkey to the skillet and let it brown for about seven minutes before transferring over to the slow cooker.
4. Add the broth around the turkey legs and then place the lid on top of the slow cooker.
5. This dish will need to cook for about seven hours on a low setting. Serve this with the parsley and enjoy.

# Chapter 7: Seafood Options the Whole Family will Love

## Coconut Shrimp

**What's inside:**

- Cilantro (.25 c.)
- Lemon garlic seasoning (2.5 tsp.)
- Thai Red curry sauce (.5 c.)
- Water (1.75 c.)
- Light coconut milk (3.75 c.)
- Shrimp (1 lb.)

**How to make:**

1. Take out the slow cooker and add in the cilantro, lemon garlic seasoning, water, red curry sauce, and coconut milk.
2. Give everything a stir before cooking on a high setting for about two hours.
3. After this time, add the shrimp to the mixture and cook for another thirty minutes.
4. Garnish with some cilantro before serving.

# Salmon Curry

## What's inside:

- Salt
- Pepper
- Turmeric (1 tsp.)
- Smoked paprika (2 tsp.)
- Bell pepper paste, red (1 c.)
- Chili powder (1 tsp.)
- Cumin (1.5 tsp.)
- Coriander (1.5 tsp.)
- Vegetable stock (.5 c.)
- Coconut milk (2 cans)
- Chopped celery stalks (3)
- Grated ginger (2 tsp.)
- Garlic cloves, chopped (6)
- Chopped onion (1)
- Salmon fillets (6 pieces)

## How to make:

1. Take out the slow cooker and add in two cans of coconut milk.
2. Add in the pepper, salt, turmeric, paprika, cumin, coriander, vegetable stock, and red bell pepper paste.
3. Stir in the rest of the ingredients, place the pieces of fish in as well, and then put the lid on top.
4. Cook this on a low setting for about two hours before serving.

# Shrimp Scampi

**What's inside:**

- Raw shrimp (1 lb.)

- Minced parsley (2 tsp.)

- Chopped garlic clove (2 tsp.)

- Olive oil (2 Tbsp.)

- White wine vinegar (.5 c.)

- Fish stock (.25 c.)

**How to make:**

1. Take out the slow cooker and add in the parsley, chopped garlic, lemon juice, olive oil, white wine vinegar, lemon juice, and fish stock.

2. Add in the thawed shrimp and place the lid on top of the slow cooker.

3. This dish will cook on a low setting for 150 minutes. After the time is up, take the lid off and serve warm.

## Asparagus Tilapia Dish

**What's inside:**

- Clarified butter (.5 Tbsp. for every fillet)
- Lemon juice (12 Tbsp.)
- Pepper
- Tilapia fillets (4 to 6)
- Asparagus (1 bunch)

**How to make:**

1. Cut out enough foil so that each fillet has a piece. Then divide up the asparagus so there is an even amount to go with each fillet.
2. Lay the fillets on the foil and sprinkle with some lemon juice and pepper. Add the butter to the top.
3. Fold the foil on top of the fish and seal up the ends. Do the same thing with all of the fillets and then add to the slow cooker.
4. Cook this on a high setting for about two hours before serving

# Chapter 8: Meat Recipes

## Pot Roast

**What's inside:**

- Pepper
- Salt
- Beef broth (.5 c.)
- Steak seasoning (1 Tbsp.)
- Quartered yellow onion (1)
- Baby carrots (1 lb.)
- Quartered russet potatoes (1 lb.)
- Trimmed chuck roast (2 lbs.)

**How to make:**

1. Slice up the roast into four pieces. Arrange the beef along with the onion, potatoes, carrot, and beef in the slow cooker.
2. Sprinkle these with the steak seasoning and pour the broth on top.
3. Place the lid on the slow cooker and cook this on a low setting for eight hours.
4. After this time is up, move the beef over to a cutting board and slice up.
5. Serve this with the juice and the veggies in the slow cooker and enjoy!

## Beef Brisket

### What's inside:

- Garlic powder (1 tsp.)
- Stevia (2 Tbsp.)
- Dijon mustard (2 tsp.)
- Worcestershire sauce (2 Tbsp.)
- Apple cider vinegar (.33 c.)
- Ketchup (.5 c.)
- Pepper
- Salt
- Chili powder (2 tsp.)
- Garlic powder (2 tsp.)
- Trimmed beef brisket (5 lbs.)

### How to make:

1. Bring out your slow cooker and place the brisket inside.
2. Take out a bowl and combine together the pepper, chili powder, and garlic powder. Use this mixture to rub the brisket on all sides.
3. In another bowl, combine together the garlic powder, stevia, Dijon mustard, Worcestershire sauce, apple cider vinegar, and ketchup.
4. Pour this sauce over your brisket before adding the lid to the top.
5. Cook this on a low setting for the next ten hours.

6. When the time is up, move the brisket over to a cutting board and slice it into thin pieces.

7. Return the sliced brisket to your slow cooker and stir in with the sauce before serving.

# Dijon Pork Chops

## What's inside:

- Chopped thyme (1 tsp.)
- Cashew cream (1 c.)
- Pork chops (4)
- Maple extract (1 tsp.)
- Minced garlic (1 tsp.)
- Dijon mustard (.25 c.)
- Chopped onion, sweet (1)
- Chicken broth (1 c.)
- Olive oil (1 Tbsp.)

## How to make:

1. Add some olive oil into the slow cooker to grease it up a bit. Then add in the maple extract, Dijon mustard, garlic, onion, and broth.
2. Stir these ingredients together well before adding the pork chops on top.
3. Place the lid on the slow cooker and cook these for eight hours on a low setting.
4. After the eight hours are done, stir in the cashew cream and top with some thyme before serving.

# Swiss Steak

## What's inside:

- Coconut cream (.33 c.)
- Minced parsley (2 Tbsp.)
- Pepper
- Salt
- Beef blade steaks (6)
- Dried thyme (1 tsp.)
- Sliced white mushrooms (1.5 lbs.)
- Sliced yellow onion (2)
- Chicken broth (.5 )

## How to make:

1. Prepare the slow cooker and then add in the thyme, mushrooms, onions, and broth.
2. When those ingredients are ready, add the beef to it and season everything with the pepper and salt.
3. Cover the slow cooker and let these ingredients cook on a low setting for the next nine hours.
4. After this time, move the steak to a platter and cover with some foil.
5. Allow the liquid to settle on the bottom of the slow cooker for a bit, and then use a spoon to move the extra fat from the top.
6. Add the parsley and the cream to the slow cooker and season with some pepper and salt.
7. Serve the steaks with some of this sauce when it is ready & enjoy!

## Lamb Steaks

**What's inside:**

- Chopped bell pepper (.25 c.)
- Chopped mint (1 Tbsp.)
- Basil, chopped (1 Tbsp.)
- Chicken broth (.5 c.)
- Lamb steaks (4)
- Pepper
- Salt
- Minced garlic cloves (3)

**How to make:**

1. To start this recipe, take out a bowl and stir together the pepper, salt, and garlic.
2. Use this mixture to rub the lamb steak on all sides before moving it over to the slow cooker.
3. Pour the broth all over the lamb steaks before adding the lid on top. Cook these for the next five hours on a low heat setting.
4. After that time is done, move the steak to a serving platter and season with some more pepper and salt.
5. Garnish this steak with some bell peppers, mint, and basil before serving.

# Chapter 9: Soups and Stews

## Turkey and Spinach Soup

**What's inside:**

- Red chili flakes
- Salt
- Cubed turkey meat (1 c.)
- Minced ginger (1 Tbsp.)
- Oregano (1 Tbsp.)
- Baby spinach (4 c.)

**How to make:**

1. Take all of the ingredients except the meat and add to the slow cooker.
2. Add in enough water to help cover up the vegetables and then close the lid on the slow cooker.
3. After seven hours on a low heat setting, turn off the heat and let it set for a few minutes.
4. Take the lid off the soup and use an immersion blender to help make the soup smooth.
5. Now, add in the turkey cubes and close the lid. Cook this for another hour on a low setting before stirring and serving.

## Sausage Soup

**What's inside:**

- Mushroom stock (3 c.)
- Red chili flakes
- Salt
- Minced ginger (2 Tbsp.)
- Cubed sausages (1 c.)
- Chopped onion (1 c.)

**How to make:**

1. Take the mushroom stock, red chili flakes, salt, ginger, sausages, and onion and add them to your slow cooker.
2. Place the lid on top and cook for six hours on a low heat setting.
3. After this time, let the soup set for a bit before opening the lid.
4. Stir everything around well and then cook for another few minutes without the lid on top. Serve it warm.

# Feisty Crab Soup

## What's inside:

- Salt (1 tsp.)
- Vegetable broth (3 c.)
- Red chili flakes
- Salt
- Minced garlic (1 Tbsp.)
- Cubed crab meat (1 c.)

## How to make:

1. Take your crab cubes and coat them with some lime juice. Let them set to the side for a bit.
2. Now, add these along with the rest of the ingredients into the slow cooker and place the lid on top.
3. Cook these on a medium setting for the next three hours.
4. After that time, take the lid off, turn down the heat setting to low, and allow the soup to simmer for a bit longer.
5. Check your seasonings to see if they are enough for you and then serve.

# Onion and Garlic Borscht

## What's inside:

- Arrowroot (2 Tbsp.)
- Coconut cream (1 c.)
- Dried dill weed (1 tsp.)
- Bay leaf (1)
- Red bell pepper paste (5 Tbsp.)
- Vegetable broth (8 c.)
- Chopped carrots (3)
- Onions and garlic (2 c.)

## How to make:

1. Take out the slow cooker and add the dill weed, bay leaf, pepper paste, carrots, vegetable broth, onion, and beets.
2. Cover the slow cooker and cook for six hours on a low heat setting.
3. Take the lid off the slow cooker and discard the bay leaf. Then bring out your immersion blender to puree the soup.
4. Mix a bit of the soup liquid with the coconut cream and arrowroot. Stir this back into the soup.
5. Cover and cook on a low setting for another 20 minutes to get the soup to thicken before ser

# PART 2

Acid reflux is one of the most common ailments affecting adults today. This is due to the notion that there are so many contributing factors and catalysts that can spawn its symptoms. As a result, educating oneself on the best ways to care for the symptoms of reflux is paramount for avoiding and overcoming them once they arise.

Evidently, a common refrain for most reflux sufferers is to avoid foods and drinks that are spicy and or fizzy. While these are certainly helpful approaches to take, you are well advised to consider approaches such as increased exercise for maintenance of overall health, avoiding certain exercises altogether if you are already suffering from severe GERD, implementing dietary changes such as limiting coffee intake, cutting back on peppermint and avoiding highly acidic foods.

But acid reflux symptoms are not caused solely by poor dietary choices alone. Indeed, smoking in excess and excess alcohol consumption are also consistent contributing factors that can induce acid reflux symptoms leading to GERD and Barrett's disease. Leveraging the knowledge presented in this book with regard to the specific dietary and lifestyle changes you must implement, along with acquiring a deeper understanding of the particular scientific reasons for acid reflux, will allow for an informed perspective so that your approach to the symptoms presented is equipped with the most up-to-date and effectual information.

When equipped with these strategies and general knowledge concerning acid reflux, you will certainly be at a distinct advantage when you are confronted by the painstaking and, at its most extreme, life-threatening, symptoms of acid reflux.

# Chapter 1: Chronic Acid Reflux & Its Serious health Implications

Acid reflux is the result of abundant backflow of acid for your stomach into the esophagus. Anatomically, when your lower esophageal sphincter (LES) becomes weakened by, among many causal factors, continually consuming a high diet, acid can flow back into your esophagus causing acid reflux. Consequently, there are numerous symptoms that are spawned by acid reflux including, most notoriously, heartburn and indigestion. While high acidity in the gut is common for everybody and is often devoid of serious health concerns if occurring on a minimal basis, serious health concerns can develop if high acidity can persist for a prolonged period of time. If left unattended and without measures of control put in place, in many instances, these health issues will lead to hospitalization or even death.In the most serious cases, chronic long-term heartburn, known as Gastroesophageal Reflux Disease (GERD), Barett's esophagus and esophageal problems can arise due to uncontrolled and unaddressed chronic acidity. Some of these most serious ailments are the remnants of years of neglecting the symptoms of acid reflux, particularly after big meals. Over time, the backflow of acid from your stomach damages your esophagus causing erosion of the layers lining the walls of the organ. This inflammation often leads to very painful swelling in esophagus called esophagitis and is accompanied by a painful swallowing feeling. In addition, esophageal ulcers are the most common ailment of an inflamed esophagus. In fact, GERD is the main cause of these ulcers in the lining of the esophagus. Moreover, painful swallowing, nausea, chest pain contribute to a lack of sleep which perpetuates many of these symptoms simplify virtue of that fact that your body is not getting the required rest to overcome these symptoms. As soon as these symptoms arise, be sure to consult a doctor too so that you can be prescribed medication to treat the symptoms before they grow into more serious, persistent conditions. Acquiring medial intervention is especially important when dealing with an ulcer; indeed, ulcers are extremely harmful to the lining of your organ and can be incredibly persistent if left unattended and given time to grow.

Even more, if your highly acidic diet remains the same as before the ulcer, this contributing factor will only enhance the growth of your ulcer and some of your other symptoms. Over time, the scarring of the lining within your esophagus will lead to scar tissue build up, thereby narrowing the esophagus altogether. Swallowing food and drinks will be made much more difficult as a result and may require a surgical procedure to expand the esophagus. These narrow areas of your esophagus are called strictures, and will likely lead to dangerous weight loss and or dehydration. Avoiding a procedure through immediate medical treatment of high acidity is clearly the preferred approach; but once these strictures block your esophageal pathways, a surgical procedure will be required.

Another common ailment of high acidity that affects many people is Barret's esophagus. Specifically, around 10%-15 of people who suffer from GERD will begin to also develop this painful condition, which results in dangerous changes in cells due to excess stomach acid. Thankfully, less than 1% of those who suffer from Barret's esophagus will actually develop esophageal cancer. If intervened early enough in the process, doctors are able to remove any of these abnormally developed cells through a procedure known as an endoscopy, whereby doctors will insert a flexible tube accompanied by a small camera into your esophagus. However, those who have GERD are at a, albeit slightly, increased risk of developing esophageal cancer. Even still, be sure to consult a doctor as soon as your symptoms reach a persistently painful level so that proactive measures and treatment can be implemented to quell your pain, and inhibit the growth of cancer cells.

If there is a long history of esophageal cancer in your family, you will be at an increased risk of developing this cancer as well, especially if you attain medical treatment after a prolonged period of time experiencing symptoms of high acidity. If you are aware of having a family history of esophageal cancer, make sure to ask your doctor for a regular endoscopy to find and mitigate the growth of improper cells. Moreover, tooth decay is a very common symptom of excess stomach acid as it wears down the outer layer of your teeth (enamel). As a result, this can lead to excess cavities and weakened teeth. In a recent study, researchers found that over 40% of GERD patients showed significant tooth decay, along with 70% of patients whose reflux had managed to reach the upper esophagus), compared to only 10% of those patients that had no symptoms of reflux. Certainly, reading about the symptoms that accompany stomach acid is disconcerting and worrisome. Nonetheless, being aware of the symptoms and knowing the early signs of their emergence will mitigate the risks of cancer and other chronic ailments like GERD and Barret's esophagus.

So, what can you do about these symptoms and potentially life-altering health concerns if you are experiencing excess stomach acid? Initially, and rather obviously, begin by assessing your diet. If you typically consume large meals, cut down your portions by at least 25%, and avoid eating right before you sleep. The latter is especially important for your digestive track as your body has to work harder to digest food whilst you are asleep and when your body's organs are supposed to be at rest. Also, limit your chocolate and coffee intake. Typically, medical professionals recommend limiting your coffee intake to only 2-3 cups per day at the most. If these levels are exceeded, your body's acidity levels will climb to healthy proportions and heighten your likelihood of acquiring the aforementioned symptoms. In the same way, excess consumption of alcohol and peppermint carry very harmful side-effects. Not mention, smoking is by far the most dangerous to many of your body's organs, especially the esophagus. Taking steps to cut back and eventually quit smoking is strongly recommended to not only avoid esophageal cancer and weakened tooth enamel, but for a bevy of other health-related reasons not directly associated with stomach acidity. When consulting a doctor to address stomach acid symptoms, you will most likely be prescribed an antacid, H2 blocker or a proton pump inhibitor (PPI); all three are available by prescription as well as over the counter.

Where GERD is concerned, there are other major factors that you should look out for. These symptoms are not specific to a particular body type or even certain foods. First, heartburn is, as mentioned, a clear indicator of GERD and is usually an only an occasional issue that is known to affect over 60 million people at least once or twice a month on average. However, for the 20 million individuals who suffer from heartburn on a chronic level through GERD, seemingly unrelated symptoms can inevitably result in numerous other health complications. You are well advised to consult a doctor if you find that you suffer frequent heartburn (two-three times per week regularly).

When you suffer from GERD, acid, food, as well as digestive juices tend to flow back into your esophagus from the pit of your stomach. Over time, this results in esophagitis, thereby leaving the king of the walls of the esophagus extremely vulnerable to additional harm through scarring, tearing and even deterioration. Additionally, while the primary symptom of GERD is heartburn, there are likely to be other symptoms that are far more difficult to diagnose for doctors and patients alike. Notably, doctors refer to a symptom known as, "silent reflux," which includes voice changes, chronic coughing, major and prolonged throat soreness, along with hoarseness. Patients may have a sustained sensation of having a lump in their throatier having the constant urge for having to clear one's throat. Another common symptom of GERD is the effect that stomach acid has on your breathing. Indeed, GERD, for instance, can heighten the extreme effects of asthma and or pneumonia. Whether or not patients have a history of lung problems personally or with regard to their family lineage, GERD can cause difficulty in breathing and persistent shortness of breath. However, treating this particular symptom is especially tricky; according to several recent studies, GERD medication, like PPIs, have been shown to increase pneumonia by directly contributing to the growth of harmful bacteria. Also, researchers have found that many prescribed PPIs suppress coughing that is needed to clear the lungs. As a result, your doctor may be forced to consider the function of your lungs when prescribing PPIs when in the process of treating symptoms associated with acid reflux.

Many people with ulcers from acid reflux tend to spit up blood and or see it in their stool. For a point of clarity, be sure to note that Esophageal ulcers are much different than stomach ulcers as they (stomach) are usually due to bacteria. Blood from esophageal ulcers, however, tend to be red or a darker purple-red color. If you find yourself having such symptoms, be sure to contact your doctor immediately. The immediate response from your doctor will likely be a schedules endoscopy mentioned earlier. In addition, you may also be prescribed acid-blocking or acid-reducing meds can treat these dangerous stomach ulcer.

An overarching common symptom of acid reflux is a lower quality of life. According to a 2004 study from Europe, whereby 6,000 GERD patients reported that their quality of life had been significantly diminished due to problems that are associated with drink, food and sleep, along with social and physical limitations. Not to mention, there can be major financial implications from having to buy an abundant amount of medications to treat the myriad symptoms of acid reflux, as well as the possible surgical procedures and endoscopy sessions that may be needed if the symptoms escalate to advanced stages. Moreover, the quality of life for patients of GERD was strikingly similar to heart-attack patients and was even lower, in certain cases, for those patients struggling with diabetes and cancer.

Generally, the healing time-frame for GERD is around 2 to 8 weeks. If allowed to persist without medicinal intervention, symptoms of GERD can inflict a considerable amount of damage. For example, reflux esophagitis (RO) can create visible and painful cracks and breaks in the esophageal mucosa. In order to fully and effectively heal RO, acid suppression for a prolonged period (roughly 3-9 weeks) is required and will likely be the timeframe advised by your doctor. Keep in mind that healing rates will rapidly improve as acid suppression increases.

Chronic stress is also a significant factor in the development, growth and. persistence of acid reflux. Our digestive system, moreover, is intricately associated with our nervous system. When stress presents itself, especially in an overwhelming or uncontrollable manner, our digestive system will then receive a lower amount of blood flow, thus causing various issues. Further, our gut bacteria are implicated in our management of stress at increasing levels, so probiotics are helpful in helping the management of this development.

# Chapter 2: The role of Fibre, Prebiotics and Probiotics

Incorporating key changes into your diet can carry massive benefits with regard to dealing with the many symptoms of acid reflux. Specifically, consuming more fiber is an excellent way to mitigate the harsh symptoms. An important point of clarity is the distinction between dietary fiber, defined as edible but non-digestible carbohydrate-based material, and insoluble fiber. Dietary fiber is mainly available in abundance naturally in many cereals, grains, plants, and vegetables as these all play a major role in gastrointestinal health. Given the importance of fiber, and its positive impact in easing the symptoms of acid reflux, many people on average are dangerously deficient in fiber. This deficiency includes both the soluble and insoluble forms of fiber. The main difference between these two forms of fiber are found in their role in digestion; insoluble fiber expedites the travel of foods through the gastrointestinal tract, while solute fibers have been shown to slow the digestion process.

While the varied and, at times, monotonous science concerning acid reflux is still in progress and remains to be settled. Nevertheless, the theoretical benefits of adequate intake of fiber include avoiding trigger foods altogether, as well as the stomach-filling "full" effect of fiber and fewer relaxation reactions of the anti-reflux valve residing between the stomach and the esophagus. Even still, there exists a persistent relationship between acid reflux trigger and the role of fiber. To elaborate, soluble fiber has been shown to induce the body to draw fluid out of already digested food, which then contributes added bulk to your meals which leaves you with a feeling of being "full" for a far more prolonged period of time. As it is commonly found within such sources as barley, peas as well as oat bran, soluble fiber does play an active role in regulating glucose levels and may even contribute to signaling the brain that the stomach is in fact full both during and after eating a meal of any size. Moreover, smaller meals can help acid reflux by refraining from overfilling your stomach. Whereas, insoluble fiber as found within vegetables and whole grains can speed up the passage of stomach contents to your intestinal tract, thereby decreasing your body's propensity for reflux.

Additionally, fatty, fried foods are typically much lower in fiber and are also frequently accompanied by the triggering symptoms of regurgitation, indigestion, and heartburn. Indeed, a fiber-rich diet like fresh fruits, vegetables, and whole-grain bread can tend to contribute to fewer instances of reflux symptoms arising. Some dietary fibers are also widely considered to be probiotics. Note the key distinction between prebiotics and probiotics: the latter refers to the specific helpful bacteria itself, with prebiotic referring to bacterial nutrients. In other words, prebiotics are nutrients which are left for bacteria to digest, or, more plainly, fuel to encourage the balanced bacterial growth within digestive organs. Here, the role of fiber in greatly improving the many symptoms of acid reflux is illuminated; this role is as a bacterial intermediary. On the whole, nonetheless, particular items in your diet tend to perform a seemingly minor role in the symptoms associated with acid reflux. Those who suffer from chronic acid reflux are strongly advised to avoid those specific foods that can aggravate painful heartburn and regurgitation; however, eliminating a broad range of food from your diet is no recommenced as it can detrimental to your overall health. Instead, you should note foods and beverages that can trigger acid reflux specifically and root them out from your diet as soon as possible

There is a tremendous amount of evidence in favor of incorporating a fiber-rich diet into your daily routine. Notably, the benefits are particular to the overall maintenance of your gut and with regard to managing the amount of harmful bacteria native to that region of your body. A study from 2004 that involved over 65,000 people revealed that fiber intake was associated with the improved perception of acid reflux symptoms. Also, this study revealed people who consumed high fiber bread were nearly three times as likely to experience relief of acid reflux symptoms compared to people who consumed bread with lower fiber content. Granted, the reasons for these results remains unknown; however, the authors of the broad study have speculated that the digestive process of fiber can also be a catalyst for enhanced muscle relaxation from the stomach through the esophagus as it tightens the anti-reflux valve.

So, what are the disadvantages of fiber in acid reflux? It is true that fiber is especially helpful when serving to ease acid reflux symptoms, excess fiber consumption has been shown to aggravate the symptoms. A study published in a medical journalism 2014 indicated that consuming a minimum of 10 grams of highly fermentable starches each day can significantly contribute to painful episodes of acid reflux symptoms. An additional study noted that nine participants who were diagnosed with GERD, those patients who consumed a prebiotic known as fructooligo also had elevated instances of acid reflux symptoms than those patients who were given a placebo.

There are many aspects to consider when striving to efficiently manage acid reflux symptoms. Among them, dietary fiber is perhaps the most important or, at the very least, the most consequential. For instance, while being excessively overweight is certainly risk factor as far as GERD is concerned, adequate consumption of healthy fiber will aid in keeping the weight at a healthy level. Excess fiber, however, causes stomach distension in may people, along with enhanced stomach pressure as well as prolonged emptying on the stomach in many cases, all of which have shown to lead to accentuated acid reflux symptoms. Medical professionals specializing in gastroenterology strongly recommend implementing lifestyle changes such as eating smaller sized meals on a frequent basis (as opposed to larger meals a few times per day), limiting overall consumption of carbonated beverages and foods high in salt content with the intent of improving the acid reflux symptoms. Note that women over the age of 50 should try to consume 25 grams per day; on the other hand, men under 50 are strongly advised to consume 38 grams of fiber each day. While consuming more laxatives is often the approach undertaken by people dealing with symptoms of acid reflux, medical professionals advise increasing your fiber content within your diet for maximized results, as well as maintaining your overall health as laxatives can take a substantial toll on your body and its digestive tract. Consuming a higher amount of fiber will strengthen your stool, keep wastes traveling more smoothly through your intestinal tract, along with preventing constipation. During this process of consuming more fibre, be sure to also ensure that you are consuming plenty of water as well; for fiber to have its absolute best effect, it is imperative that your body remain as hydrated as possible to make sure that waste moves smoothly along your intestinal tract rather than building up due to rigidity.

A good source of probiotics and fiber is yogurt, which carries "good" bacteria helpful for overall maintenance of gut health. A healthy gut is paramount for an efficient and well-functioning intestinal tract and digestive system. Prebiotics and probiotics are, essentially, analogous to food for the bacteria in your stomach; bananas, corn, and whole wheat are additional food sources that are high in prebiotics. Moreover, one of the most beneficial aspects of a fiber-rich diet is the notion that high-fiber foods help control your cravings for snacks. Certainly, high fiber diets can help you lose weight as it displaces other calories for overall maintenance of health.

Guarding against illness, fiber-rich diets will also lower your chances of developing major gut-related illnesses such as diverticulitis. This condition, pockets in the walls of colon trap waste as opposed to moving it along. While doctors remain unsure of the direct catalyst(s) for the illness, consuming a high-fiber diet moves waste fervently along through your system. Along with diverticulitis, a high-fiber diet also eases and prevents irritable bowel syndrome— which has also been linked to acid reflux, albeit a rarer, more extreme symptom. Nevertheless, the most common symptom of acid reflux— heartburn— is quelled by a fiber-rich diet.

Probiotics are becoming increasingly linked to the management of the symptoms associated with acid reflux and alleviating these issues. For a more technical explanation, as we are already aware that probiotics are an effective way of balancing the gut bacteria inside of our bodies, they also help combat against a bacterial infection knows as, H. pylori. This bacterial infection usually originates in childhood. This bacteria, found in the stomach, can alter the environment around them through reducing the acidity levels so that they can survive for longer periods of time. By penetrating the lining of the stomach, thereby remaining hidden and protected by the mucous membrane so that the body's immune defenses cannot reach them. In addition, these bacteria tend to secrete an enzyme called urease, which converts urea to ammonia. The presence of ammonia in this instance is significant because it reduces the stomach acidity around the specific area where the bacteria is found. Coincidentally, it is this lower stomach acid that is often mistaken— by doctors and patients alike— for acid reflux. Can probiotics help combat H. pylori? Well, many medical researchers believe that probiotics can, in fact, help battle this bacteria in several key ways. For one, probiotics are believed to strengthen the protective barrier against H. pylori by producing antimicrobial substances, along with competing against H. pylori for what is known as adhesion receptors (space on the lining of the stomach). Also, it is believed that probiotics assist in stabilizing the gut's mucosal barrier. Many researchers even argue that the production of relatively large amounts of lactate is another inhibitory factor of H. pylori due to the possibility that it could lower the H. pylori urease. Not to mention, probiotics may also be effective in modifying inflammation levels by interacting with the epithelial cells that are responsible for managing the secretion of inflammatory proteins in the gut.

Depending on the particular cause of your acid reflux, probiotics can be incredibly useful for alleviating the painful symptoms. Probiotics can be taken in conjunction with an antacid without worry of the antacid overtaking the positive benefits of the probiotic. More importantly, your approach should be to uncover the root of your acid reflux and adjust medical intervention accordingly. Of course, you doctor plays a huge role in this process, especially in diagnosing the specific cause of your acid reflux; still, it is your responsibility to seek medical expertise so that you can tackle the root of the symptoms as opposed to addressing the individual symptoms as they arise. Being aware of the triggers in both the food and drinks that you consume, managing your stress levels regardless of how often they fluctuate, and finding the specific levels of acid within your stomach are critical steps to address the symptoms of acid reflux. More likely than not, the best method of dealing with your symptoms will be to implement a diverse approach that incorporates a range of approaches rather than relying solely on medical intervention.

# Chapter 3: Understanding the role of proteins, carbs, AND fats in healing acid damage

In recent years, there have been increasing reports concerning the benefits of a low-carb diet in healing the damage induced by acid damage. This may seem counterintuitive given the notion that the standard treatment for GERD includes the *removal* of certain foods that increase acidity in the stomach, for example, tomato sauces which are believed to be contributing causes of excess stomach acidity. Also, as mentioned in chapter 1, the removal of coffee, alcohol, smoking, and peppermint are other dietary and lifestyle changes that ease GERD symptoms. Additionally, researchers have found that diets with a higher amount of carbohydrates can significantly elevate symptoms of acid reflux. Whereas, a low-carb diet has also been shown to reduce symptoms of GERD. While many health researchers and medical experts have expressed concern over the exceptionally low proportion of daily calories from fat and protein in low-carb diets, as wells calorie levels being considerably lower in these diet than recommended. Nevertheless, the effects of gastroesophageal reflux disease have been shown to be significantly reduced after implementation of a low-carb diet. For a case in point, following a 2001 research study in which 5 individuals with diverse ranges of GERD symptoms and across the age spectrum, engaged in a low-carb diet, each of the 5 research participants showed significant relief of symptoms. Granted, throughout the duration of the study, which spanned 8 months, 3 of the 5 research participants also reduced their coffee intake concurrently.

The concurrent reduction of coffee, coupled with lower intake of carbohydrates, was shown to be effective in reducing symptoms such as heartburn and stomach pain. Interestingly, while coffee reduction was a contributing factor, observations from a few of the participants revealed that exacerbating foods such as coffee and fat are less pertinent when a low-carb diet is strictly followed. In other words, when implementing a low-carb diet, the effects of classic factors like coffee and fat intake are vastly diminished even if their consumption is not significantly reduced. So, whether or not you choose to reduce coffee and fat intake significantly, you are likely to reduce most GERD symptoms by solely undertaking a low-carb diet. Therefore, the logical conclusion to draw from these findings is that a low-carb diet is a significant factor for reducing the symptoms of acid reflux. This conclusion gains even more credibility when considering the propensity for high-carb diets to aggravate GERD symptoms.

In addition to lower carbohydrates, lean sources of protein and healthy fats are beneficial for reducing symptoms associated with acid reflux. Lean proteins found in eggs are a great addition to your diet for reducing acid reflux symptoms; however, they are a problem for many people due to elevated cholesterol. If eggs are an issue for you, be sure to consume only egg whites and refrain for consuming higher fat yolks—which have been shown to elevate GERD symptoms. Moreover, as high-fat meals and fried food typically descries LES pressure thereby delaying emptying of the stomach and boosting the risk of acid reflux, it is in your best interest to choose lean grilled meats, as well as poached, baked or broiled meats. Boosting proteins, in the way, will also provide benefits for your overall health as well. Also, complex carbohydrates, as found in rice, whole grain bread, couscous and oatmeal carry excellent benefits for reducing GERD symptoms and easing any scarring that may already be present in the walls of your esophagus. Specifically, brown rice and whole grains add valuable fiber your diet. Root vegetables such as potatoes are excellent sources of healthy carbohydrates and easily digestible fiber. Remember to refrain from incorporating too much garlic and onion while preparing your meals, which are can commonly irritate the esophagus and stomach lining.

Along with proteins and complex carbs, incorporating healthy fats has great benefits for easing GERD symptoms and other symptoms accompanying acid reflux. A type of nutrient, fat is high in calories but certainly a necessary component of your diet. Keep in mind, however, fats can vary and they do not all have the same effect on your body. On the whole, you are well advised to avoid consuming a high amount of saturated fats as typically found in dairy and meat, along with trans fats found in processed foods, shortening and margarine. As a replacement, unsaturated fats from fish and or plants are recommended; some examples of monounsaturated fats include sesame, olive, canola, sunflower, peanuts, seeds and nuts, as well as butter. In addition, examples of polyunsaturated fats include such oils as safflower, corn, flaxseed and walnut, fatty fish such as salmon and trout, along with soybean.

Some other helpful tips for reducing acid reflux symptoms include chewing gum, as long as it is not spearmint- or peppermint-flavored. Chewing gum increases the amount of saliva production in your mouth and also reduces the amount of acid in your esophagus. While alcohol consumption has already been mentioned in earlier chapters, research suggests that some people begin to experience extreme symptoms after only one drink; if you fall into this category, be sure to experiment with your levels to uncover what amount is best for you. Additionally, during and after each meal, particularly bigger meals, be sure to remain aware of your posture. Generally, it is a good idea to sit up while you are eating and avoid lying flat on your back for at least hours post-meal. Standing up and walking around the room after a big meal can help encourage the flow of gastric juices in the right direction. Further, avoiding eating big meals before bed can help you refrain from overloading your digestive system while you sleep. Digestion increases the overall amount of gastric acid that is present within your stomach. When laying down, LES's ability to inhibit stomach contents from traveling through the esophagus decreases significantly. When operating concurrently, excess stomach acid and remaining in a reclined position for an unexpended period of time create an abundance of acid reflux symptoms. On the whole, consuming a large meal for less than 3 to 4 hours prior to bed is generally not advisable for those suffering from persistent GERD symptoms; however, the timing of these symptoms can certainly vary depending on the individual.

In a 2017 research study on the benefits of healthy dietary changes versus drug intervention, researchers studied the effects of dietary changes to a type of reflux known as laryngopharyngeal reflux or LPR. This reflux is essentially triggered when pepsin, a digestive enzyme from the stomach, reaches the sensitive tissues in the upper section of the digestive tract.

Symptoms like throat clearing and hoarseness are common with pepsin in the throat and or upper part of the digestive tract. In the study, the researchers had participants suffering from acid reflux switch to a Mediterranean diet and consuming significantly more water, thereby neutralizing excess acid. In this particular study, participants avoided classic triggers such as coffee, peppermint, alcohol, fatty and spicy foods, chocolate and soda. Another set of participants were given pharmaceutical drugs to ease GERD symptoms.

After a six week timeframe, participants of the study reported a greater percent of declines in their GERD symptoms as those participants that had used drugs to address the symptoms. Granted, the study did not elaborate on the particular ways in which that the diet and increased water consumption eased the symptoms; nonetheless, the Mediterranean diet incorporates eating mostly plant-based fruits and vegetables. In addition, the increased water can mitigate pepsin's acidity levels in the throat. As mentioned, fruits, vegetables and water are great methods of reducing acid reflux and GERD symptoms. With this in mind, the positive benefits experienced by the study's participants is not surprising in the least.

Adjusting your diet for GERD does not require removing all of the foods that you typically enjoy eating. Instead, a few simple changes to your diet if more than enough to address the uncomfortable symptoms of GERD. Your aim in addressing the GERD symptoms should be to create a well-rounded, nutrient-based diet that incorporates a variety of foods that include vegetables, fruits, complex carbs, healthy fats and lean sources of protein. Healing acid reflux damage is made significantly easier when starting with dietary changes that add healthy and diverse foods. Coupled with medical intervention (if required), healthy dietary changes can carry great benefits for healing scarring in your esophagus and stomach, as well as symptoms such as heartburn, bloating and even tooth decay.

# Chapter 4: Exercise to reduce acid reflux

When GERD symptoms escalate and you are still in the early stages of implementing dietary changes to address acid reflux symptoms, exercise can be a great option for reducing the symptoms. When GERD symptoms begin to arise, high-impact physical activities like running, skipping rope and jumping exercises. If you are overweight or obese, a weight loss of 10% has been shown to reduce GERD symptoms like heartburn, bloating and reflux. A self-reported analysis study of individuals experiencing GERD symptoms fund that those who reduced their Body Mass Index (BMI) by 2 kilograms or 4.4 pounds or more, along with the circumference of their waist by 5cm or more has improved their GERD symptoms significantly. In contrast, there are also certain exercises that can induce reflux by opening the lower esophageal sphincter (LES) during workouts such as heavy lifting, stomach crunches, or other high impact exercises. When the LES opens, stomach acid travels up into the esophagus causing heartburn.

There are some common sense tips concerning exercise for managing GERD symptoms. First, this twice about how much and what you are eating prior to starting your exercise routine. Obviously, less food in your stomach is ideal. If you are too full, you should wait at least 1 to 2 hours before initiating your exercise routine. This will allow for food to pass fro your stomach through to the small intestine. With less food in your stomach while exercising, it is significantly less likely that you will experience the painful and annoying symptoms of acid reflux such as heartburn and bloating. Next, you should choose the food you consume with thought and, in some instances, caution. Generally, you should avoid foods that trigger GERD symptoms (choosing complex carbohydrates is advised). Your stomach does metabolize these foods much faster than others through a process known as gastric emptying.

Moreover, diabetics should avoid high fat and high protein foods before exercise due to being more susceptible to experiencing slow gastric emptying. Experts also suggest adjusting your workout if you suffer from frequent GERD symptoms. Starting at a slower pace with workouts that put less strain on your body like controlled walking and controlled weight training in either a sitting or standing position is strongly recommended. Whereas, high impact, high-intensity workouts like running, rowing and cycling and induce acid reflux. Additionally, acrobatic workouts and gymnastics can also disrupt stomach contents. The key is to avoid exercises that jostle the LES and reflux, these are typically positions that put your body in awkward positions like being upside down defying gravity in one way or another.

A great exercise that carries tremendous benefits for improving and relieving acid reflux symptoms and digestion is yoga. One particular study from 2014 found that six months of yoga significantly reduced acid reflux and stomach bloating, along with improved esophagitis. Again, however, try to avoid positions that heighten GERD symptoms. If any of these "lifestyle" changes fail to improve your GERD symptoms during exercise, be sure to consult your doctor about being prescribed medication for acid-suppression. And, of course, engaging in a constant exercise routine is not only very beneficial with regard to improving your GERD symptoms, but also for the maintenance of your overall health.

# Chapter 5: How to live a reflux free life?

As you may have already noticed, acid reflex can be induced by an abundance of factors ranging from diet, bad habits, poor sleep hygiene, and many other factors. Clearly, it isn't just as simple as cutting out bad habits and instilling a series of great dietary and lifestyle changes. But whether you are able to successfully implement these changes or not does not, thankfully, hinge on strict adherence to a stringent diet or eliminating some of your favorite guilty habits. But before you can begin to consider stepping into a reflux-free life, you should be cognizant of the stages of reflux and recovery.

Firstly, almost everyone who suffers from GERD begins with normal LES and little to no reflux. The severity level of GERD, therefore, more than likely correlates to best with the overall degree of damage inflicted upon the sphincter. Note, however, that this is not easy to determine. Normally, the amount of damage to your sphincter correlates with the overall severity of acid reflux symptoms. This severity is most often determined by the volume, frequency, and duration of reflux episodes. In turn, these factors will correlate with GERD symptoms such as regurgitation and heartburn. If you are diagnosed with GERD, your strategy for addressing the symptoms and eventually overcoming them should first be to containment. Unfortunately, damage to your LES caused by GERD cannot be reversed by drugs and is permanent. Nonetheless, many patients of GERD have been able to live with these symptoms and with functionality despite damage to the sphincter. Changing simple lifestyle habits, such as sleeping and eating, can significantly decrease and prevent severe reflux episodes in spite of damage to your sphincter.

In Stage 1 of GERD, known as Mild GERD, most adults currently have minimal damage to their LES and tend to experience mild GERD occasionally. Most often, the adults are left with either tolerating occasional heartburn or will have to use over-the-counter acid suppressive medications from the onset of symptoms through its subsequent stages. Typically, when taking drugs to address the symptoms, quality of life for patients is not affected because the medications are very effective in suppressing symptoms. If you choose to take medication to address symptoms, make sure that you are also cleaning up your diet. If you continue to consume trigger foods and beverages, like coffee and certain sauces, for example, the benefits you garner from medication will be minimal and your recovery will be prolonged if not inhibited altogether. Replacing these meals with smaller, leaner meals that do not pose a threat to inducing symptoms of GERD is recommended. This will ease heartburn and lessen the damage to your sphincter.

In stage 2, known as Moderate GERD, symptoms are far more difficult to control and use of prescribed acid-suppressive drugs will be needed. In this stage, reflux is accompanied by symptoms that are far more intense than stage 1. Therefore, medicinal intervention is needed to mitigate the damage and pain caused by these symptoms. Still, many symptoms in this stage can be managed by using acid-suppressive drugs for prolonged periods of time. Keep in mind that over-the-counter medication can provide insufficient relief; whereas, prescription strength medications are needed in order for you to manage GERD symptoms effectively. Additionally, stage 3, or, Severe GERD, can result in a very low quality if life and is generally considered to be an extremely serious problem by medical professionals specializing in GERD. Because prescription grade acid-suppressive drugs and medicinal intervention usually do not control symptoms, regurgitation is frequent. In Stage 3, it is entirely possible that complications associated with erosive GERD are present. Lastly, stage 4, or,  reflux-induced esophageal cancer, is quite obviously the most serious stage. The result of numerous years of severe reflux, nearly 16% of all long-term reflux sufferers progress to this extremely advanced stage. Due to the long-term reflux, the esophagus' lining has been heavily damaged, thereby resulting in a high degree of cellular changes. Also, stage 4 is the stage that involves the pre-cancerous condition called Barrett's esophagus and or an even more severe condition called dysplasia. Granted, these conditions are not cancerous. However, they are capable of raising the risk of developing reflux-induced esophageal cancer. Accordingly, at this stage, common GERD symptoms are likely to also be accompanied by a strong burning sensation in the throat, chronic coughing, and persistent hoarseness. A narrowing of the esophagus, or strictures, will also be present in this stage, and can also be characterized by the sensation that food is sticking to your throat. However, this is only a feeling associated with strictures. Notably, this symptom is also caused by esophageal cancer. Keep in mind that stage 4 GERD can only be diagnosed by a medical professional through an endoscopy and from an intrusive biopsy of cells retrieved from the lower esophagus.

A 30-day recovery plan for GERD symptom can be easily broken into weekly steps. In the first week, you will presumably be trying to lean off of the medication that you have been prescribed. A reversion plan of this nature should take into account a variety of approaches that incorporate dietary changes, exercise routines, sleep schedules, and other lifestyle changes. Drinking more tea and water is strongly recommended throughout your 30-day reversion plan, as long as the tea is not peppermint-flavored. Also, in your first week of recovery, be sure to get as much sleep as possible, in conjunction with eating 2 to 3 hours before you sleep. A meal should also be incorporated throughout this entire 30-day stretch. This plan should include egg whites in the morning, instead of coffee switch to tea for your caffeine fix. For lunch, whole grain bread with lean meat- chicken or turkey preferably- with light sauce and a bevy of vegetables. Moreover, dinner should include a balanced meal that provides nutrients and foods that will not induce heartburn. Remember, this meal should be consumed a few hours before bed so that your body has time to properly digest the food. Also, be sure to refrain from lying directly on your back after your meal; as mentioned, this will induce acid reflux symptoms like heartburn and excess bloating.

In week 2, in keeping with the consumption of nutrient-rich food and water consumption from the previous week, you should begin an exercise routine of you have been devoid of routine prior to week 2. A consistent exercise routine will help maintain overall health so that your body has excess strength and energy to overcome the wear and damage inflicted from GERD symptoms. Also, a consistent exercise routine will boost your metabolism so that you can burn off excess unhealthy fats and complex carbohydrates that can cause strain to your body and induce reflux symptoms. In the third week of your 30-day revision plan, you can slightly increase the size of your meals. Still, make sure that the overall size of your meals remain relatively small, with only slight additions where you may see fit. By week three, your exercise routine, water consumption, and sleep habits should be starting to feel more routine and many of reflux your symptoms will begin to diminish. Moreover, leading into week 4, your diet should continue to incorporate nuts, vegetables, fruits, tea, and other plant-based foods and drinks to expedite the healing process. However, the final week of your 30-day recovery plan is vital for sustaining the progress that you have presumably made since the start of the month. It is vital because you must ensure that you do not get too comfortable in your routine that you allow for gradual decline back into the habits that spawned your acid reflux. Pushing through this final week will augment your progress and solidify your path to living a reflux-free life. Specifically, with regard to your diet, you can incorporate the following fruit and vegetable smoothie recipe. Smoothies and healthy shakes are an excellent meal replacement option for optimal health and recovery from acid reflux

Add 2 scoops of frozen berries into a 400ml cup

Add 2 scoops of spinach from a 250ml scoop

Add 2 tablespoons of Chia Seeds

Add 2 tablespoons of hemp hearts

Add 1 tablespoon of peanut butter

This smoothie should be blended with water to ensure that it is not excessively thick.

# PART 3

Whether you're just considering Bariatric surgery, trying to figure out if you'd be a good candidate, or if you have the date set for surgery and you want to know what to expect and how to prepare, want to know about post-op care and recovery, or how to maintain your body after surgery, this can help anyone from the beginning steps all the way until months after. You'll find out what the requirements are for surgery and if you can qualify, the different kinds of procedures and the pros and cons of each one, how you'll need to prepare and what diet restrictions you'll have after surgery. This book will also include foods that you can and can't eat before and after surgery along with a meal guide for after your procedure. This will be the beginning of a whole new lifestyle for you so congrats on taking the first step to making that change!

# Chapter 1: What? Who? And Why?

What is Bariatric surgery? By definition, Bariatric surgery is a surgical procedure performed on the stomach or intestines to induce weight loss. Weight loss is achieved by wrapping a gastric band around the stomach to reduce its size or by re-routing the small intestine to a small stomach pouch. The procedure causes weight loss by restricting the amount of food the stomach can hold. The most common types of procedures are Gastric Bypass, Gastric Sleeve, Adjustable Gastric Band, and Biliopancreatic Diversion with Duodenal Switch (BPD/DS).

- Gastric Bypass
  - o This is done by dividing the top part of the stomach, then dividing the first portion of the small intestine and attaching it to the top piece of the divided stomach.
  - o Pros: On average you'll lose 60%-80% of your excess weight, restricts the amount of food you can consume, can lead to increased energy, positive changes in gut hormones that enhance satiety and reduce appetite.
  - o Cons: It's a more complex operation compared to the other procedures, which could result to more complications, it could lead to long-term vitamin/mineral deficiencies (particularly in Vitamin B12, iron, calcium, and folate), typically a longer hospital stay is required compared to other procedures, requires following your doctor's dietary recommendations, and could lead to life-long vitamin/mineral supplementation.

- Gastric Sleeve

- o This procedure is done by removing 80% of the stomach. The new stomach holds much less than the normal stomach so there's much less calories being consumed.

- o Pros: It restricts the amount of food that your stomach can hold, induces significant weight loss in a short amount of time, and it does not require any foreign objects or rerouting the food stream, normally a short hospital stay (about 2 days), and causes changes in gut hormones that suppress hunger, reduce appetite and improve satiety.

- o Cons: The procedure is non-reversible, there is a possibility of having long-term vitamin/mineral deficiencies, and there is a higher chance of an early complication rate.

- Adjustable Gastric Band

  - o This involves putting an inflatable band around the upper portion of the stomach. This creates a smaller stomach pouch above the band.

  - o Pros: Reduces the amount of food that can go into the stomach, typical weight loss of about 40%-50% of your excess weight, it does not involve any cutting or rerouting, requires a much shorter hospital stay compared to other procedures (usually around 24 hours or you can even be released the same day), this procedure is reversible, has the lowest rate of early post-op complications, and has the lowest risk for vitamin and mineral deficiencies.

  - o Cons: This procedure has the highest rate of re-operation, it requires sticking to a strict post-op diet and going to your post-op follow up visits, dilation in the esophagus can result if you overeat, you may experience mechanical problems with the band, procedure requires a foreign device to remain inside of your body, a higher percentage of patients fail to lose up to 50% of excess body weight, less early weight loss, and slower weight loss compared to other procedures.

- Biliopancreatic Diversion with Duodenal Switch (BPD/DS)
  - o There are two parts to this procedure. First, a portion of the stomach is removed, leaving a tube shaped stomach. Then, a large portion of the small intestine is bypassed.
  - o Pros: Average weight loss is about 60%-70% of your excess weight at a 5 year follow up which is much greater than other procedures, it is the most effective procedure against diabetes, causes changes in gut hormones that improves satiety and reduces appetite, reduces fat absorption by 70% or more, and it also allows patients to eventually eat more "normal" meals.
  - o Cons: There is a higher risk compared to similar procedures, requires a longer hospital stay, requires a very strict compliance with follow up visits and dietary/vitamin supplementation recommendations, and guidelines are critical to avoiding serious complications such as protein and vitamin deficiencies.

If you have been considering Bariatric surgery, I hope the list above has given you some things to consider when you think about which procedure would be right for you. Depending on which procedure you have done that can affect how long you're in the hospital, your recovery time and how much weight you lose after the surgery.

Who would be a good candidate for Bariatric surgery? If you are considering surgery, then there are a few things you need to ask yourself first. One of the first questions you need to ask yourself is what is your BMI? If you have a BMI over 40, then most organizations would say that weight loss surgery is a reasonable option for you, but you must be healthy enough to sustain surgery. To give you an example, if your height is 5'5" then your BMI would be 40 if you weighed 240 ½ pounds. The next question you should ask yourself is do you have any weight related medical conditions? In some cases, certain medical conditions may help qualify you for surgery, but others might make you not able to withstand the procedure. If you have a BMI of 35 or over, you may qualify for surgery if you have at least one obesity related medical condition such as Type 2 Diabetes, hypertension, gastrointestinal disorders, heart disease, non-alcoholic fatty liver disease, osteoarthritis, lipid abnormalities, sleep apnea and other respiratory disorders.

Why should you consider Bariatric surgery? Most people that are considering having these procedures done or already have had them done have tried other weight loss options and have not been successful with them. If it's at all possible to avoid surgery, then you should go with that option since all procedures are not without their own risks. Some examples of a non-surgical option to losing weight would be diet and exercise, a support group or a partner who will motivate you, supplements or weight loss medication. If you haven't tried any of these options, then you may not qualify for surgery.

We now know what Bariatric surgery is and the different procedures that are available. You should pick the procedure that will best fit your needs and consider all the risks that comes along with each procedure, along with the benefits. Some procedures have higher risks than others and some can make you lose a higher amount of weight in a shorter amount of time. You should consider both the risks and benefits when choosing one. Once you've weighed your options and you have figured out if you would be a good candidate and why you want the surgery, that will better help you in finding out which one would be the best option for you. Once you know which procedure you will be doing, we can move on to how you can prepare for you big day.

# Chapter 2: Preparing for Surgery

This surgery is a big step into your new lifestyle. In order to prepare you'll have to make a few changes. First, if you are a smoker then it will be required that you stop smoking before your surgery. This will reduce the risk of some complications after surgery. If you don't quit smoking before surgery it can cause breathing problems before and after the procedure, and you'll have a higher risk of developing pneumonia. Smoking also slows down your blood flow, which means you won't heal as fast. On top of that making your recovery time much longer, that also means you are at risk of infection for a much larger period of time than you normally would have been. It's recommended that you quit smoking at least a week in advance. But even quitting just one day in advance can decrease your chances of complications, although the earlier the better. You will also need to stick to any medications your physician has prescribed you along with any dietary restrictions that were given to you. Unless given a diet to follow by your doctor, here is a diet that you should follow at least 3 weeks before your surgery.

- You should be eating at least 60 grams a day of protein.
- Eliminate all refined sugars and reduce carb intake.
- Eat healthy fats, avoid bad kinds of fat.
  - Healthy fats: Avocado, fish, nuts, olives, etc.
  - Bad fats: Butter, vegetable oil, fast food, cake, etc.
- Avoid high calorie foods.
- 48-72 hours before surgery you should be on an all liquid diet. Do not consume any solid food.

- The night before your surgery you should stop consuming all liquids and food. This allows the surgeon to operate without any interference.

  o You also may need to stop taking certain medication before surgery. Inform your doctor of any medication you are taking so they can tell you what is and isn't safe to be taking before surgery. Medications you may need to stop taking include arthritis medication, NSAIDS (nonsteroidal anti-inflammatory drugs such as Tylenol, Aspirin, Ibuprofen, Naproxen), and any anticoagulants (Enoxaparin, Clopidogrel, Dipyridamole, Ticlopidine, and Warfarin). Any medication that acts as a blood thinner should be removed from your diet to remove the risk of complications during surgery.

  o Other planning may be needed depending on the length of the hospital stay and your recovery time. These can vary based on which procedure you are having done. You may want a family member, close friend or spouse to stay with you at the hospital or at home with you for support once you are released. It is also a good idea to make home and/or work arrangements since you will be recovering for a few weeks.

You will also need to mentally prepare yourself for surgery and for life after. You need to find the root cause of your weight gain. Is it because of a health issue? Stress? Is it because of depression or a food addiction? Many people who are obese whose cause is not related to a health issue may have problems with food addiction. It is imperative that you know food addictions not dealt with after surgery can have dire consequences. You can severely harm yourself if you continue the food addiction after you have the surgery. The reason this is so important is because when you eat large amounts of food it can cause your stomach to rupture. This can happen with a normal stomach so your chances of having your newly, much smaller stomach rupture rapidly increase. Having this procedure done will not make food addictions go away. That is a lifestyle change that only you can make. You must want to change, surgery or no surgery. If you don't, you will have severe consequences to deal with.

Preparing for your procedure may be a little tough but it's preparing you for your new lifestyle ahead. Since you'll be recovering for a little while after surgery remember to take care of any responsibilities you may have over the next few weeks and to not have anything to eat or drink for the 24 hours leading up to the surgery. It may be hard to do but keep your goals in mind and let them motivate you.

# Chapter 3: Your Surgery Day!

After all the time you've spent preparing, it's finally here. It's time to get your surgery! The morning of your procedure there are still a few last preparations. Any medications you are still taking should only be taken with a sip of water, anything that could be lost or is going to be taken off should be left at home, and wear something comfy. You're going to be here for a while, so you should make yourself comfortable. You've been eating a pretty restrictive diet lately and have consumed nothing at all the past 24 hours. On top of that you're probably feeling nervous. Don't freak out, it's completely normal to feel this way but knowing what to expect can help you to relax. When you arrive at the hospital, you'll sign some paperwork and get checked in, then you'll be taken back to an examination room. Here you'll do your pre-op physical, EKG (a process that records electrical activity of the heart) and have some blood/lab work done. Then a physician will come out to go over your procedure and this is when any questions you may have can be asked and answered. You'll be given an I.V. and then you'll wait until someone comes to get you. When they come to get you to bring you back for surgery you will be taken back to the operating room on a stretcher. Your family/friends that are there with you will go wait in the waiting room until you are done with your procedure. Before your surgery starts your anesthesiologist will give you a medication and you'll go to sleep.

A nurse will notify your family when your surgery is complete and the surgeon that performed on you will speak to them in the waiting room Depending on the type of procedure you had done, you'll either wake up on a stretcher or a hospital bed. You will always have an R.N. available to you and if you need any pain medication then there will be a button for you to push. Discomfort after surgery is normal but report if you feel any sudden/severe pain or shortness of breath. Some common complaints are shoulder pain, soreness on the left-side abdominal area, nausea, constipation/diarrhea, gas pain, weakness, and fatigue. Keep in mind this is just a guideline. This is a researched example to give you an idea of what to expect on the day of your surgery.

Congratulations, you made it! I'm sure you're excited and will want to know how much weight you can expect to start losing. You should ask your doctor, but your results can be varied depending on multiple factors. This depends on which procedure you had done, how much you weigh now, and how you take care of yourself from here on out will all contribute to your weight loss results. Most people lose about 60% of their excess weight after gastric bypass surgery. Now that you're done with your surgery and are now recovering, you can learn about post-op care.

# Chapter 4: Post-op Care

Before we talk about post-op care, I'm going to include some side effects that you might experience after surgery and include if they are just a common side effect, or if they can seriously harm you so you'll know what to look out for.

- Constipation (common)
  - o This is very common after weight loss surgery. Inform your doctor and they will instruct you on what to do.
- Gallstones (common)
  - o Up to 50% of patients will develop gallstones after weight loss surgery because it develops when you lose a lot of weight in a short amount of time.
  - o 15%-25% of people will need surgery to remove their gallstones after gastric bypass surgery.
  - o Gallstones can also cause nausea, vomiting and abdominal pain.
- Blood clots in your lungs (serious)
  - o This is rare, happening only 1% of the time but is still a possibility.
  - o Although this can be life threatening, blood thinning drugs can usually prevent blood clots. Frequent activity can also prevent it.
- Bleeding in stool (serious)
  - o This can appear reddish or black and is very serious. Inform your doctor immediately.

84

- Dumping Syndrome (common)
  - This can happen if you eat meals that are high in sugar after weight loss surgery.
- Wound infections (common)
  - This can happen up to 3 weeks after surgery.
  - Symptoms include redness and warmth, pus, and pain from the wound.
  - Requires antibiotics and could possibly need surgery.
- Leaks (serious)
  - Rare, but serious.
  - Can occur up to 5 days after surgery.
  - Symptoms include abdominal pain and feeling ill.
  - Call your doctor if you think that you are experiencing this.

Post-op care is very important, especially for weight loss surgery. As previously mentioned, you can severely harm yourself by not following certain guidelines. Dietary guidelines are extremely important to follow, and they are critical to your health, recovery and success with your weight loss journey. Vitamins and minerals are also very important to take because they will give you the nutrients that you need after your surgery. Most procedures also cause vitamin and/or mineral deficiencies so taking them will help to prevent that. It would be a good idea to incorporate some exercise into your routine, daily physical activity is important. It's recommended that you get 30 minutes each day. There are also support groups if you want some extra help to stay motivated. These groups are for people who have had weight loss surgery and would like to share advice, thoughts and concerns, ask questions, and overall give support. If you aren't comfortable with a group maybe you can find a family member or a close friend that is interested in doing this journey with you and you can motivate each other to reach your goals.

Although your surgeon will probably give you a list of recommended foods, some of the food items for a Bariatric surgery post-op diet are tea, sugar-free, non-carbonated beverages, non-acidic juices, broth (chicken, beef, vegetable) cottage cheese, oatmeal, and cream of wheat. There is a diet progression which you MUST follow. This is extremely important, if you try to eat something that is too solid too soon then you could possibly rupture your stomach. The diet progression goes clear liquids, full liquids, pureed foods, soft foods, and then finally solid foods. It could take 4-12 weeks for you to go through the entire progression. How quickly you go through it can depend on the type of surgery you had, speed of recovery, and your body's natural tolerance to the food progression. During the clear liquid diet phase, you can only drink liquids that are see through. This includes tea, water, diluted fruit juice that is non-acidic, protein fruit drinks, sugar-free gelatins, and artificially sweetened non-carbonated drinks. Once your body can handle clear liquids, you can move onto the full liquid phase. In this phase you can have protein shakes, skim milk, low-fat cream soups, low-fat yogurt, sugar-free gelatin, and sugar-free pudding. The next phase is pureed foods. This is soft food blended up to have a smoother consistency, to make it easier for your stomach to handle and does not have any chunks in it. The type of food that is included in this has a pretty large range because it doesn't have to originally be soft since it's getting blended.

Next is the soft food phase and this is when you can start eating actual food again, but it needs to be easy to chew. This can include steamed vegetables, soft fruit, pasta, and oatmeal. Even though your eating soft foods it can still be hard on your stomach. Make sure your food is mushy and you've thoroughly chewed it before swallowing. It will probably take you 30-60 minutes to finish a meal if you are chewing properly. I know this may seem tedious, but it's very important that your food is completely chewed so that it is easier to digest. It may tire you now while eating but you'll thank yourself later when your stomach can digest what you've eaten. The last phase is the solid food diet. Once you can normally eat soft foods again you can move onto this phase. You should slowly add solid food to your diet and more and more will be added gradually so that your digestive system can get used to the solid food. You should still be chewing slowly and thoroughly even at this phase. Once again I know it may seem like you can handle it but your stomach is very sensitive right now and even when you move up to solid foods, especially when you move to solid foods, you'll need to chew thoroughly and slowly to take it easy on your stomach. Along with the dietary progression you should be following dietary guidelines as well so that you are getting the nutrition that your body needs. You should choose healthy foods that are low on fat and high in protein. Remember to drink plenty of fluids throughout the day but avoid drinking with meals. One of your biggest concerns is going to be making sure you're eating enough protein. Protein is not something that the body replenishes. For women, the daily requirements are 50-60 grams. For men, the requirements are 60-70 grams. You may need to take protein supplements to meet your daily requirements after surgery.

Something that you'll have to be slow and consistent with is your fitness after surgery. It's important to keep you body healthy and this will help you work towards your goal. After surgery if you are planning on exercising, take it very SLOW. There are countless people that tried to do too much, too soon after their surgery and ended up bedridden for a week or more. This will set you back quite a bit as far as your fitness goals are concerned so if you really want to keep progressing then you will be extra careful to not go too far. In the days immediately following your surgery, the medical team will be telling you to walk as much as you can. You should spend the first few days at home getting up out of bed and walking around the house. Any physical activity is good, get up and walk around if you're bored or to watch T.V. It seems like it's pointless but it's really not. Any kind of exercise will increase the blood flow in your body. By moving around, this tells your brain that your muscles are being used and this will burn calories. The only thing that you are able to consume right now is a protein shake, so you aren't consuming any substantial amount of calories. When your body burns calories and they aren't being replenished then it will have to pull those calories from somewhere and start dipping into your fat reserves, this burns fat! At a few weeks out form your surgery you can start doing easy exercise. Such as leg lifts, shoulder rolls, any sitting exercises, and you can continue walking too. You can just increase the distance. Once you're about a month down the road from your surgery, you'll be able to crank it up a notch. Some exercises you should be able to do at this point are water aerobics and cycling. After a few more months you should be able to move onto strength training. This includes yoga, squats, and lunges. You can try going to the gym or do a workout from home. Start out with something easy and work your way up. If you choose to go to the gym you can start out with a smaller pair of weights and make a workout routine. If you choose to stay at home, it can be as simple as having a yoga mat and some resistance bands.

With any post-op care, whether it's eating or exercising, please take it slow! It may seem like things are progressing way too slowly, but your body needs this time to get used to doing things again after all it's been through.

# Chapter 5: Life After Surgery

The first few weeks after surgery you'll probably be a little sore and be on an all liquid diet. You'll start walking around even if it's for 5 minutes at a time. You shouldn't try to do anything more physically demanding than that. Even a few months after surgery you'll still need to take it easy. You'll be eating more solid foods at this point and able to do more physically. At 6 months after surgery you'll have had a bit of weight loss. If you had gastric bypass surgery, then you will have lost 30%-40% of your excess weight. With gastric band surgery you lose about 1-2 pounds a week, so at this point would be anywhere from 25-50 pounds lost. One year after surgery you will have lost a significant amount of weight. The most dramatic changes happen within a year of your surgery. You are likely to your goal weight. With gastric banding you will have lost 100 pounds. If you haven't lost this amount it's important that you find the cause and make sure you are doing everything you can to contribute to your weight loss.

There are some changes you'll need to make with your personal life too after surgery if you wish to be successful with your weight loss journey. You'll need to tell your friends and family that it's very important for you to eat healthy from now on and stick to your smaller portions. It's much easier to stick to a healthy lifestyle when you have the support from everyone around you. But it can be that much harder if they don't. If your spouse, friends and family are still eating unhealthy and large portions then that can be really difficult to keep up with your healthy lifestyle. It's even possible that some people in your life might be jealous of you and might try to make you feel bad when you start to lose weight and they are still overweight. You should surround yourself with a group of people that support you and make it easier for you to live your new, healthy lifestyle. Losing weight can have a lot of impact on the relationships in your life. Hopefully for the better, but not always. How your relationship with your significant other if affected can depend a lot on how the relationship was before surgery. Did you have a good relationship? Was it not so good? If it was a bad relationship, they may have made you feel bad for being obese or maybe they liked your old weight and don't want you to change. If this is the case, they may become controlling and overly jealous when they see you losing weight. If you had a good relationship, then it should only strengthen your bond. If your S.O. decides to get healthier with you then that's great! If you have children then this choice will affect them too, but for the better! If you have a younger child, then you will help them develop healthy eating patterns and get used to eating healthy foods. If you have an older child, maybe even one that is overweight themselves, then you can help them make the changes earlier on in their life that you are now.

# Chapter 6: How to Maintain Your Body and Stay in Shape

You'll have to learn how to take care of your new body. Not just right after surgery, but for the rest of your life. You'll have to be consistent in eating healthy and exercising if you want to stay in shape, you're going to have a whole lifestyle change! To stay consistent with working out, you should find a workout routine that works for you. Don't try to make yourself do something that you don't like to do. If you aren't a runner, try swimming. If you don't like lifting weights, try calisthenics. Find something that you can see yourself enjoying and progressing in. Plan your workout for the next few days in advance or every Sunday/Monday plan your workouts for the week ahead. You'll need to make a workout plan that you'll stick with. Set simple and easy to reach goals the first time around. Don't try to accomplish too much or you could hurt yourself or give up too early when you don't finish what you planned to. I know you're excited about losing weight and you want to get started, but you are more likely to lose less weight by planning to do more than you can actually accomplish. It's great to have big goals and you should always strive to progress and push past your limits to reach your new goal, but when you bite off more than you can chew you can't swallow! In other words, it's very easy to get discouraged in the beginning if you set impossible goals for yourself. It may take some time to see results in the beginning and that can be really hard to deal with. You're putting in so much work and you don't get to see any results yet. Believe me, if you push past this hump you WILL see results and by then you will have developed a habit eating healthy and working out. It will be so much easier to remain consistent once you do this. You've overcome the hardest obstacle, it is now a habit for you, and you've started to see results! Seeing the results that you've worked so hard for is the best motivation that you could receive.

Keeping a healthy diet is another goal you'll want to make sure you're reaching. Planning your meals ahead of time is a great way to avoid sneaking in snacks, overeating and binging an unhealthy meal. It takes the guesswork out of cooking and it'll probably save you from splurging at the grocery store. I would suggest planning your 3 big meals everyday and then also prepare for 2 healthy snacks a day. One in between breakfast and lunch, and one in between lunch and dinner. For your meals you should come up with an entrée, and for your sides and snacks you should make an approved healthy list to pick from. This list can of course grow if you find any snacks or sides you would like to try that are healthy. It's your choice if you wish to only prepare for the meal or if you would like to meal prep. Meal prepping is helpful because you don't have to put any thought into what you eat after it's prepped for the week because they are completely planned out, cooked, and ready for you to grab when it's time to eat. But if you like to cook or just don't want to cook all of your meals the next few days or week then you can stick to only planning what you're going to eat. You'll still have to make your food, but this is still helpful by taking the guesswork out of what you're going to eat. You shouldn't have any snacks after dinner because you are probably winding down for the day which means you aren't using as much energy from your body as you would in the middle of the day.

Calories put into your body that aren't used will be stored and then turned into fat. Stick to liquids after dinner that way if you feel snacky you can drink some tea or water and you won't be putting very many, if any, calories in your body but your stomach will feel fuller.

Once you get started in your new lifestyle you will eventually need to progress past what you're doing now. Set new goals the same way you did your first ones. This time you are more acquainted with what you can accomplish which will allow you to set goals that will push you, but not set a goal that is unreachable. Although you should set goals that are realistically within your reach, you should never let anything get too easy and never let yourself get bored. That can go for more than just working out. You should try new things and create new challenges for yourself. Goals don't have to only be fitness related, they can be anything that helps to improve any part of your life. Your goals could include starting a new happy or progress in your job. There are so many things that we can do with life, you should never get bored! If you don't know what to do, that itself could be your goal. To go out and discover what you like. Maybe you have a creative side you never knew about. You could start writing, drawing, painting, or try out photography. Maybe you want to meet new people and make friends, or maybe you want to travel. There is so much out in the world to do that there should never be a reason to be bored. This is a great way to have a happy and healthy lifestyle before or after surgery. Staying busy and doing things that you love with people you care about can help depression, prevent overeating and unhealthy eating since you are staying busy, all of these things will help you overcome obesity.

Surgery or not, a big step in staying healthy and fit is consistency. It's going to be very hard for your body to lose weight if you aren't keeping up with your workouts and eating healthy. Pick a meal plan and a workout routine that fits your wants and needs and works with your schedule. Since your whole day is already planned it takes out any of the guesswork. You have a whole plan laid out you just have to go out and do it. Since you were productive, you'll feel happy and accomplished at the end of the day.

# Conclusion

The lectin-free diet is one of the best options for you to go with to reduce inflammation, give you more energy, and help you live your best life. It can help you by reducing the amount of lectin that you naturally eat in your meals, and it won't take long for you to see the great benefits.

This guidebook took some time to explore the lectin-free diet and what it means to your health. It is a simple idea, one that you can easily implement into your daily routine without having to make many changes. Just change up some of the foods that you eat, add in some more exercise, and you are going to see some amazing results.

If you are dealing with issues in your digestive system, if you have a leaky gut syndrome, or you are dealing with a lot of unexplained inflammation, it may be time to take a look at the amount of lectin that you are consuming. This guidebook will provide you with all of the information that you need to get started on the lectin-free diet today!

The next step is to begin implementing the various methods of relief repented within this book so that you can immediately address the symptoms of acid reflux before they take root. Addressing the symptoms, in this manner, will allow your body to fight off disease like GERD and Barrett's disease as soon as possible rather than at a later time when your body is significantly weaker. Keep in mind that the best method of addressing your symptoms is to consult a medical professional. In this way, you can begin to implement the strategies presented in this book with guidance from a qualified medical professional.

Given that your acid reflux is likely to exist on a ranging spectrum and will most definitely be different for every individual, this book provides methods of addressing your symptoms and ailments in a manner that is applicable and helpful for whichever stage of the reflux you are experiencing. What's more, the 30-day recovery plan is a great way to ensure that your symptoms are staved off for good once you can utilize medical intervention. If, for instance, you are prescribed drugs to mitigate your symptoms, be sure to use the methods outlined in this book in conjunction with the prescribed amount of medication that your doctor has instructed.

Where your health is concerned, being prepared and informed is critical to seeing that you successfully overcome the ailments that are affecting you.

That is precisely why this book is of value. After reading, you are now informed about the intricate aspects of acid reflux and should feel extremely prepared as you move forward in addressing these symptoms.

So now you know all about Bariatric surgery. The different kinds of procedures and how they differ, how to prepare for it and what recovery will be like. If you are just starting out and trying to get information, I hope this helped you and once again congrats on taking the first step to a new and healthier life. If you are preparing for surgery, I hope this has helped you with your preparations and can make you feel more secure knowing what to expect on the day of your procedure. If you are currently in recovery, then this should have helped you with your diet and physical restrictions and what you are capable of doing right now.

This book should also have given you an estimate of how much weight you can expect to lose from each type of procedure. Please keep in mind that any weight loss surgery can only help you to lose weight. You must be the one who wants to change and follow through with your plans. Surgery is not going to change your lifestyle, habits, addictions or any other cause of your obesity